Keto Copycat Recipes

Quick and Easy Cookbook for Making Your Favorite Restaurant Keto Dishes at Home

Willy Nelson

The information in the following pages is broadly considered a truthful and accurate account of facts and as such, any inattention, use, or misuse of the information in question by the reader will render any resulting actions solely under their purview. There are no scenarios in which the publisher or the original author of this work can be in any fashion deemed liable for any hardship or damages that may befall them after undertaking information described herein.

Additionally, the information in the following pages is intended only for informational purposes and should thus be thought of as universal. As befitting its nature, it is presented without assurance regarding its prolonged validity or interim quality. Trademarks that are mentioned are done without written consent and can in no way be considered an endorsement from the trademark holder.

Summary

Introduction

Going out to dinner with friends, family, and loved ones is among the greatest things in the world. Enjoying these moments of relaxation and sharing is very nice. But at what cost? Sometimes these dinners come at very high prices and are not affordable for everyone.

Do you ever wish that you could enjoy some favorite meals from your favorite restaurants without having to order takeout or visit the restaurant all the time?

People recognize that they will feel more comfortable consuming at home; However, If they don't know how to prepare their favorite meal, the food's high quality will not be as right now. Well-considered copycat recipes are the answer to that question.

Eating out at an expensive eatery can be quite tricky on your wallet and will make your finances even more difficult. If you want to save money because of your steady income, you can use a famous clean and very cheap copycat recipe book. You will be amazed at how the methods work and how they got the real taste and appreciation of your favorite pricey dish. You can even use it in all activities and sports. Likewise, you can now bring home the kitchen of your favorite restaurant with the famous copycat recipe's useful source and be the chef to prepare tons of your favorite gourmand recipes. Once you have eaten and eaten a selected dish, you will be surprised and proud to find a trendy, delicious meal and become a professional chef.

Whether you need to prepare a dinner for the whole family or have fun with co-workers and best friends, with copycat recipes, you are sure to serve an unforgettable meal to please your family and friends.

Recipes that simulate the same taste, including your favorite meal's flavor. Because it replicates the recipe, it is therefore called a copycat. The famous copycat recipes are recipes that you can cook at home.

1. French Toast

Serves: 3

Prep Time: 5-Mins

Cooking Time: 5-Mins

Ingredients:

8-slices of Texas toast or sourdough bread

1-cup of milk

2-tablespoons of sugar

4-teaspoons vanilla extract

2-pinches of salt

Butter and syrup for serving

4-eggs

Method:

Beat the eggs, milk, sugar, vanilla, and salt together in a large bowl. Heat a griddle or skillet over medium heat. Spray with nonstick cooking spray. Dip each sandwich in the egg mixture and let it soak for 25-30 seconds on all sides. Place the slices on the baking sheet or skillet and cook for 2-3 minutes on all sides or until golden brown. Serve with butter and syrup. Enjoy!

Nutrition:

Calories: 252

Carbs: 33 g

Protein: 11 g

Fat: 7 g

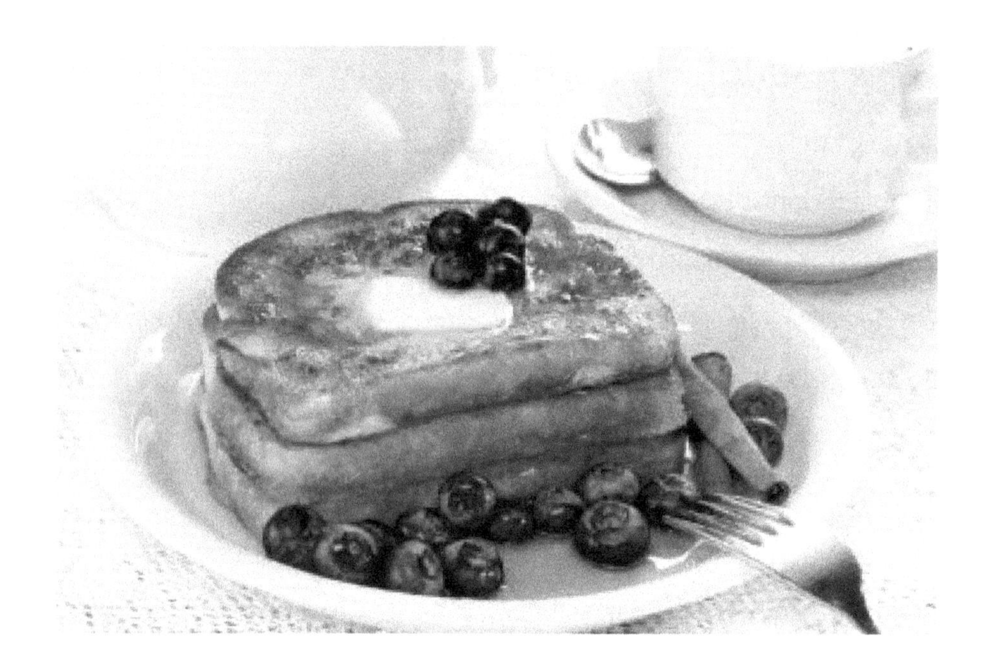

2. Turkey Devonshire Sandwich Like Armstrong's

Serves: 3

Prep time: 10-Mins

Cooking Time: 15-Mins

Ingredients:

Cheese sauce

4-tablespoons of butter

4-tablespoons of flour

1 cup of chicken stock

8 oz shredded cheddar cheese I recommend a spicy cheddar, Tillamook

1/4 cup Parmesan cheese chopped sandwich

Cooked 5-slices of bacon

4-slices of Italian bread lightly toasted

4-slices of tomato

1/2-pound turkey breast Paprika

1 cup of whole milk

Method:

Preheat the grill. Melt butter in a medium saucepan and sprinkle with flour. Cook the butter and flour aggregate for about a minute over medium heat until the meal starts to smell nutty. Add 1 cup of chicken stock and 1 cup of milk and stir until thickened. Add the sauce with Cheddar and Parmesan cheese, stir until the cheese melts. Remove the pan from the hot burner and occasionally stir, as the sandwich is formulated to keep your skin from growing on the apex of the sauce. Sandwich mounting Toast the bread. Make a slice by installing a pie pan, a slice of toasted bread, turkey, and then tomato. Spoon the cheese sauce over the sandwich. Sprinkle with a few peppers on top. Mix the cheese sauce with bacon slices. Roast until brown starts with cheese. Enjoy!

3. Honey-Cinnamon-Sweet Potatoes

Serves: 2

Prep Time: 10-Mins

Cooking Time: 5-Mins

Ingredients:

4-sweet potatoes

Honey-cinnamon butter

2-cups butter softened

2-tablespoons brown sugar

1-teaspoon ground cinnamon

¼-cup of honey

Method:

Heat the oven to 375 ° F. Wash and prick the sweet potatoes and wrap them in foil. Bake the potatoes for an hour or until completely soft. Meanwhile, mix all the ingredients for the butter. Cut the sweet potatoes open and use a fork to fluff the flesh. Add a dollop of butter to the steaming potato and serve. Store leftover butter in the refrigerator. Enjoy!

Nutrition:

Calories: 167.3

Carbs: 27.4 g

Fat: 53.9 g

Protein: 17.2 g

Sodium: 367 mg

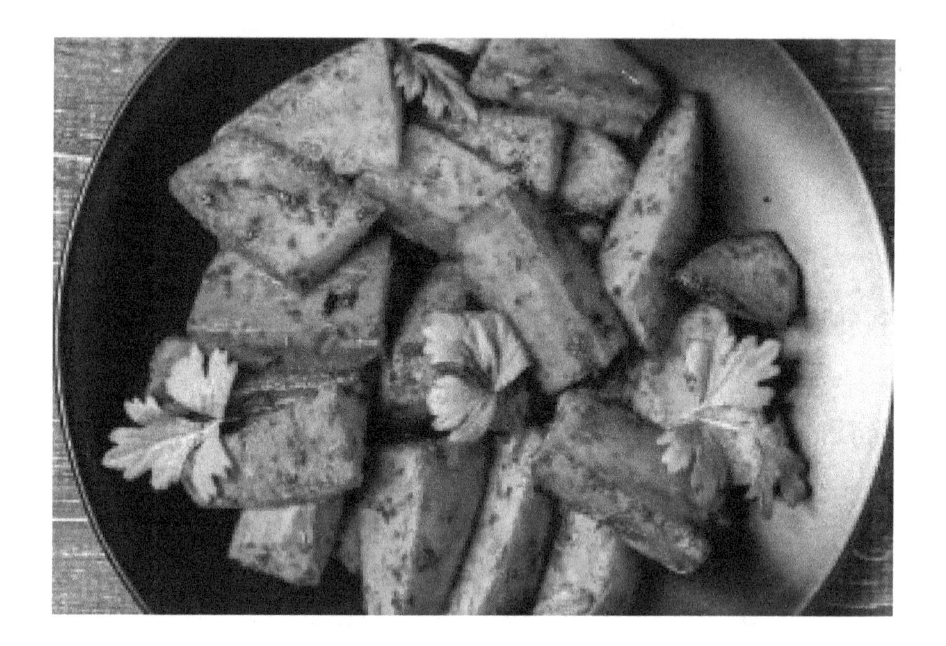

4. Eggrolls Of Southwestern Chile

Serves: 2

Prep Time: 10-Mins

Cooking Time: 5-Mins

Ingredients:

2-possibilities are very vegetable oil

1-chicken skinless, boneless, half cut

2-tablespoons finely chopped green onion

2-tablespoons min Red bell pepper

⅓ cup of corn buns

¼ cup black beans, fried and drained

2-tablespoons from chopped spinach, thawed and drained

2-common things you can see

½ tablespoon ground beef for parsley

½ teaspoon ground cumin

½ teaspoon of chili powder

1-pinch of ground cayenne pepper

5 (6 inch) flour tortillas

1 liter for deep

Add salt

Method:

Rub 1-tablespoon of vegetable oil over the chicken bread. In an interval of medium heat, cook the bird in step with the side for about 5 minutes until the flesh is now not pink and the juices are clear. Remove from heat and set aside. Heat the last 1 tablespoon of vegetable oil in a medium saucepan over medium heat. Stir in the green onion and purple pepper. Cook and stir for 5 minutes, until tender. Choose a color and mix in one plan and the other. Mix in some, black is, spinach, jalapeno peppers, parsley, cumin, chili powder, alt, and cayenne pepper. Boil and stir for five minutes, and it will usually be mixed and soft. Leave it and stir More Jack chese cheat in or that it is more. Wrap tortillas in a clean, slightly wet cloth. Microwave on high for about 1 minute, or until warm and pliable. Spoon even amounts of the combination into each dish. Meet the ends of things, then the whole combination. Secure with toothpicks. Arrange in a medium bowl, cover with plastic, and place in the freezer. Freeze for at least 4 hours. Take a large deep skillet and warm oil for frying up to 375 levels F (one hundred ninety stages C). Fry the frozen, filled tortillas every 10 minutes, or until dark golden brown. Let them drain on kitchen paper before serving. Enjoy!

Nutrition:

Carbs: 21.8 g

Protein: 13.6 g

5. Cheesy Walkabout Soup

Serves: 2

Prep Time: 15-Mins

Cooking Time: 15-Mins

Ingredients:

6-tablespoons butter, divided

2-large sweet onions, thinly sliced

2 cups low-sodium chicken stock

¼ teaspoon ground black pepper

2-chicken stock cubes

3-tablespoons flour

1 ½ cup whole milk

A pinch of nutmeg

¼ cup of Velveeta® cheese, cubed

¼ teaspoon salt

Method:

Melt half the butter over medium heat in a large saucepan or Dutch oven. Add the onions. Cook, occasionally stirring, until the onions are transparent but not brown. Add the chicken stock, black pepper, and stock cubes. Mix well and cook over low heat. Melt the remaining butter in a separate pan. Add the flour and salt and cook, constantly stirring, until smooth and light brown. Gradually beat in the milk and cook over medium heat until very thick. Mix in the nutmeg. Add the béchamel sauce to the onion soup mixture, next to the Velveeta cubes. Stir gently over medium heat until cheese has melted and everything is combined.

Nutrition:

Calories: 260

Total fat: 19 g

Carbs: 13 g

Protein: 5 g

Fiber: 1 g

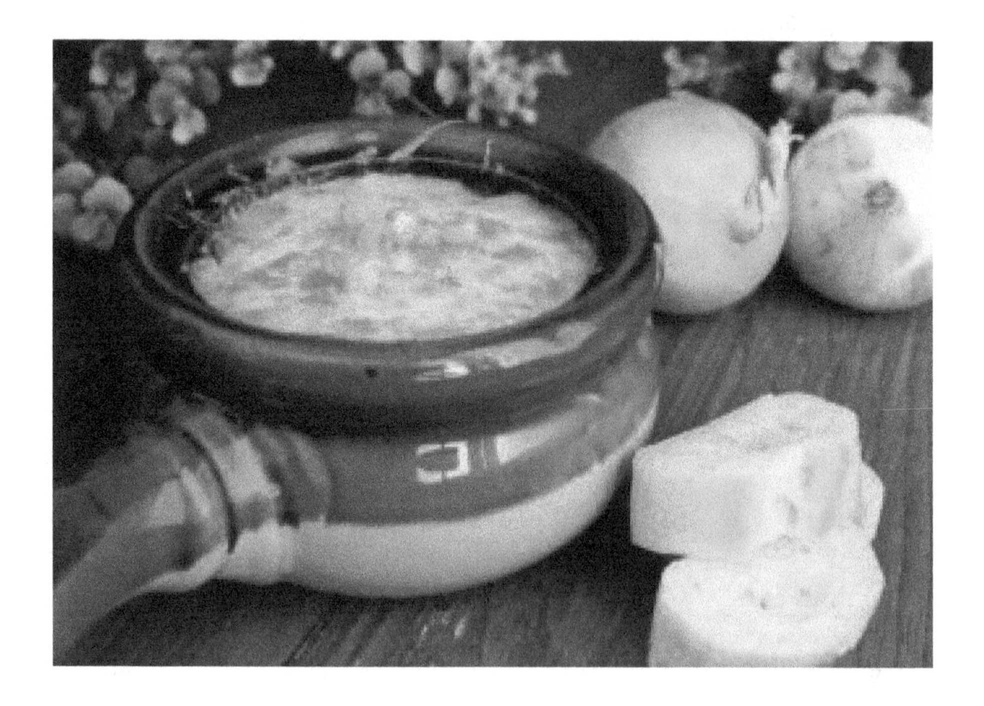

6. Boston Market Mac N 'Cheese

Prep Time: 15-Mins

Cooking Time: 10-Mins

Serves: 3

Ingredients:

8-tablespoons unsalted butter (1 stick)

1/2 cup of flour

1-teaspoon of salt

1/4 teaspoon black pepper

1/2 teaspoon dry mustard

8 ounces of American cheese

1/2 cup of blue cheese

1/2 cup of cheddar cheese

Cooked 8 ounces of semolina rotini pasta

4-cups of milk whole

Method:

Heat the oven to 400 degrees. Melt the butter over medium heat and add the flour, salt, pepper, and mustard. Beat until done and prepare for 30 seconds. Add in the milk in 1-liter increments until soft. Add to the cheese and beat until completely melted. Add to the pasta and stir. Pour into a baking dish and bake, also for 20 minutes. Enjoy!

Nutrition:

Carbs: 34 g

Protein: 17g

Fat: 29 g

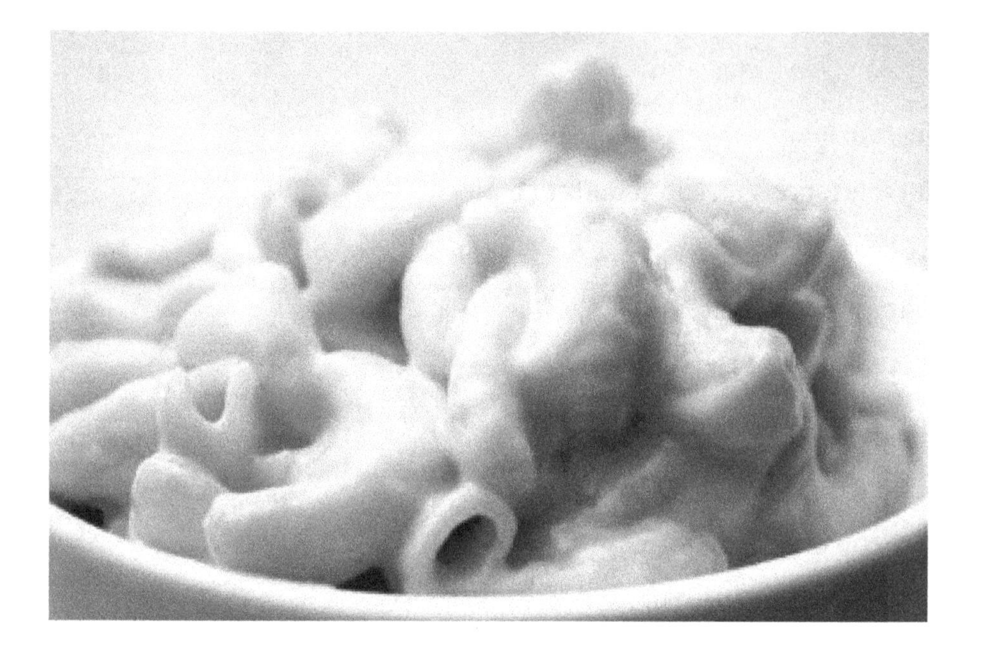

7. Cracker Barrel's Double Fudge Coca Cola Chocolate Cake

Prep Time: 12-Mins

Cooking Time: 7-Mins

Serves: 2

Ingredients:

Cake:

Cooking spray with non-stick coating

½-cup unsalted butter

½-cup vegetable oil

3-tablespoons unsweetened cocoa powder

1-cup Coca Cola

2-cups all-purpose flour

2-cups granulated sugar

1-teaspoon baking powder

½-cup buttermilk

1-teaspoon of pure vanilla extract

2-eggs

½-teaspoon salt

Glaze:

½-cup unsalted butter (1 stick), softened

3-tablespoons of unsweetened cocoa powder

6-tablespoons of Coca Cola ™

4-cups of powdered sugar

1-teaspoon of pure vanilla extract

Method:

Preheat oven to 350 ° F. Coat a large 9 x 13-inch rectangular baking pan with non-stick cooking spray. Add the butter, oil, chocolate, and Coca-Cola to a pan. Bring to a boil. Add the mixture to the electric mixing bowl. Add the sugar, flour, salt, and baking powder. Beat on medium speed until well blended. Add one egg at a time. Add buttermilk and vanilla. Beat until well blended, and the cake batter is smooth. Transfer the prepared batter to the pan and spread it evenly. Place in the oven and bake for 40 minutes. Prepare the frosting while the cake is in the oven. Beat the butter with an electric beater to cream. Add 6-tablespoons of Coca-Cola, chocolate, and vanilla. Beat until well blended. Add the granulated sugar in steps of 1 cup at a time. Beat until the icing is smooth and fluffy. Remove the cake from the oven. While the cake remains hot, spread the chocolate icing evenly over the cake. Let cool before covering with plastic parchment paper and place in the refrigerator until ready to serve. Serve with a scoop of vanilla ice cream, if desired. Enjoy!

Nutrition:

Calories: 845

Carbs: 81 g

Total fat: 49 g

Protein 23 g

Sodium: 1652 mg

8. Peanut Butter Sauce

Serves: 2

Prep Time: 12-Mins

Cooking Time: 7-Mins

Ingredients:

2-tablespoons of butter

1-cup heavy whipping cream (you can use half and a half)

1/2 cup of corn syrup

1/2 teaspoon of salt

1-cup of smooth peanut butter is recommended

1-teaspoon vanilla

1/2 cup of sugar

Method:

Add heavy cream, corn sauce, sugar, salt, and herb peanut butter in a saucepan over medium heat, melt the butter. Stir continuously until the mixture is clear. Put the sauce in the fridge and then add vanilla. Store in the refrigerator over the sauce. Enjoy!

Nutrition:

Calories: 324

Carbs: 33 g

Protein: 7 g

Fat: 19 g

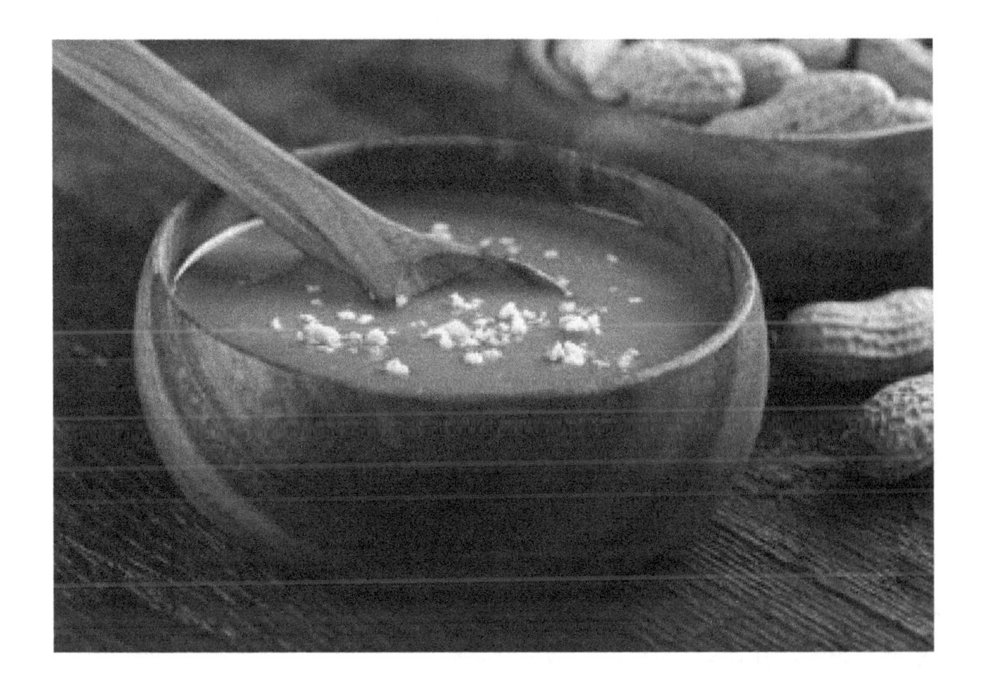

9. Coconut Shrimp

Serves: 4

Prep Time: 30-Mins

Cooking Time: 35-Mins

Ingredients:

16 large shrimps, peeled and deveined

½ cup cornstarch

½ cup all-purpose flour

1-teaspoon salt

½ teaspoon cayenne pepper

2-tablespoons vegetable oil

1-cup ice water

2-cups short shredded coconut

Vegetable oil for frying

Dipping sauce with honey marmalade

¼ cup honey

2-tablespoons mustard

½ teaspoon cayenne pepper

¾ cup orange marmalade

4-drops Tabasco® or hot sauce

Method:

Rinse and pat the shrimp dry. Mix the ingredients for the honey marmalade sauce and keep it refrigerated. In a mixing bowl, combine the cornstarch, flour, salt, and cayenne pepper. Stir in the 2-tablespoons of oil and drinking water. Mix to make a batter. Heat the oil to 350 ° F. Divide some of the shredded coconuts in a shallow bowl. Dip the shrimp into the batter one at a time, then press them into the coconut. Bake in small portions for 3-4 minutes, until golden and cooked through. Serve warm, with one side of the dipping sauce. Enjoy!

Nutrition:

Calories: 767.3

Carbs: 57.4 g

Fat: 52.9 g

Protein: 17.2 g

Sodium: 367 mg

10. Mexican Pizza

Serves: 2

Prep Time: 20-Mins

Cooking Time: 10-Mins

Ingredients:

1 pound ground beef

1-packet of taco seasoning

3/4 cup of water

1 cup of vegetable oil

8-flour tortillas (taco size)

1 (10 oz)-can of enchilada sauce

2 cups of grated Mexican cheese mix

sliced tomatoes

sliced green onion

sliced olives

sliced green onions

1-can (15 oz) of beans

Method:

Preheat the oven to 400f. Brown the minced meat and crumble it in a large frying pan. Drain extra fat. Place cooked beef lower back in the skillet, add the taco seasoning packet, water, and stir. Bring to a boil, reduce heat and simmer until thickened. Heat the oil in a large frying pan over medium heat. Add tortillas (at a specified time) and cook for 3-4 minutes (free-flying) until done. Continue with the rest of the tortillas. Put aside. Meanwhile, heat the beans in a microwave-safe bowl. It will make it less complicated to unfold the benefits in the first place. On each tortilla, have a little more of the available dishes. Then sprinkle with some ground red meat. Place every other tortilla on top. Spread over tablespoons of the enchilada sauce on top. Then put a few grated slices of cheese on top of the sauce. Continue to assemble the rest of the pizzas. Place the pizzas on a solid non-stick baking tray and bake for about 8-10 minutes until the cheese has melted. Serve with your favorite toppings! Enjoy!

Nutrition:

Carbs: 34 g

Protein: 27 g

Fat: 24 g

11. Hash Brown Casserole

Prep Time: 15-Mins

Cooking Time: 55-Mins

Serves: 12

Ingredients:

1-bag (30 ounces) of frozen hash browns, thawed

½ cup butter, melted

1-can of chicken soup

1-small onion, chopped

1-pound cheddar cheese, shredded (divided)

½ teaspoon of black pepper

1-cup of sour cream

1-teaspoon of salt

Method:

Preheat the oven to 350 ° F. Prepare a baking dish by greasing the edges or spraying with nonstick cooking spray. In a large bowl, combine the onion, chicken soup cream, pepper, and all but 1 cup of grated cheese. Mix in the sour cream until well incorporated. Add the melted butter and hash browns. Stir to mix. Pour into the greased baking dish. Bake for 45 minutes or until bubbly, then sprinkle the remaining cheese on top and bake for an additional 5-10 minutes or until the cheese has melted. Enjoy!

Nutrition:

Calories: 90

Total fat: 3.5 g

Saturated fat: 2 g

Cholesterol: 10mg

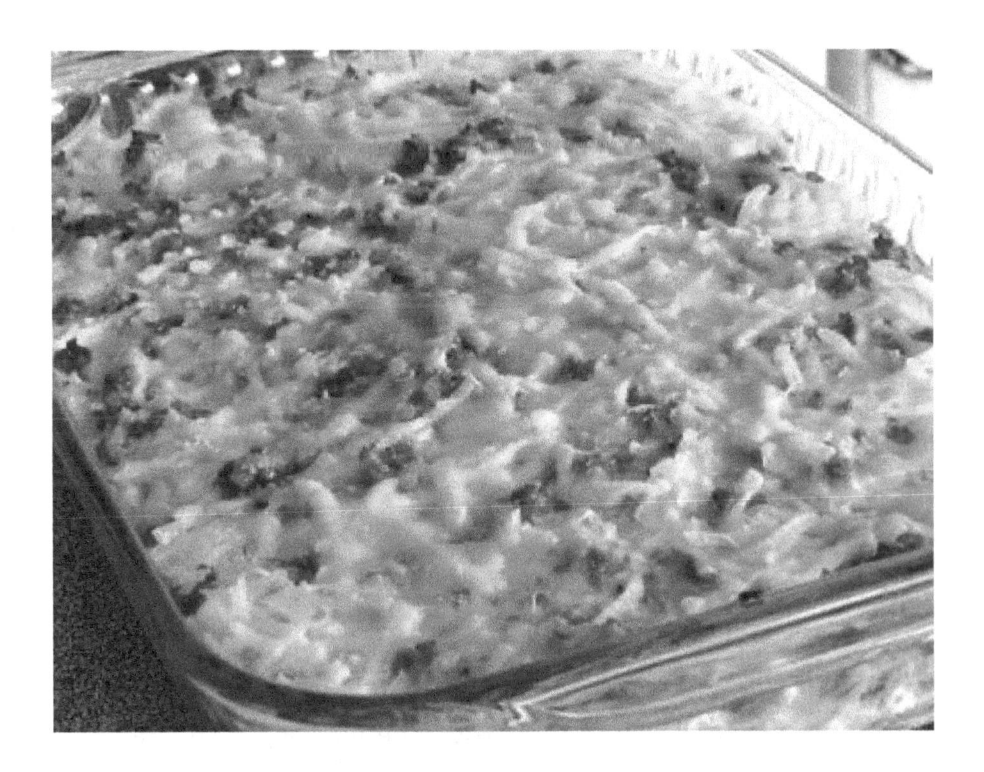

12. Sonic's Signature House Burger

Serves: 2

Prep Time: 20-Mins

Cooking Time: 25-Mins

Ingredients:

1 1/2 cups Tater Tots

1 pound ground sausage

1/2 pound bacon

6-ounces american cheese

4-tablespoons ml, divided use

10-eggs

1/2 cup of shredded Cheddar chese

1-jalapeno pepper disappears

6-flour-tortilla

salt and pepper

Method:

Preheat the oven to 350 degrees. Spray a baking sheet with nonstick cooking spray and place the Tater Tots on the baking sheet. Bake for about 22 to 25 minutes. While the potato kids are in the oven, cook the sausage in a skillet over medium heat until well browned. Pour the sausage over a paper towel and cover with another paper towel to retain the heat while still preparing breakfast. You can prepare the bacon for dinner in the same pan in which you chose the sausage. Remove the baking sheet from the pan and let it dry later. Sonic serves their burrito with a different sauce. Cut the 6 oz of American cheese and place in a small pot over low heat, and place 2- tablespoons of milk. Melt the next, often occurring mixture, and a certain one will produce a different result. Once the cheese sauce is formed, turn off the burner and remove the pan on the stovetop, the residual heat will retain the sauce liquid while you cook the eggs. In a medium bowl, integrate the eggs with the ultimate 2-pieces of milk. Spray a little with non-stick coating, about medium heat egg and milk combination. Now you need to season eggs with a pinch of salt, and a pinch of black pepper. Start things gently as they can. As soon as they are no longer off the world. Make tortillas about 60 times to make them and lay eggs while they cook. When they are done, discard the heat. Heat tortillas for about 60 seconds to make them warm and pliable. Place these over the tortillas using the eggs, sausage, potato cakes, bacon, and cheese sauce. If you need a few pieces of cheese, it looks like the blackberries do too, and if you want, sprinkle a bit of Chedurr cheese on the blackberry. If desired, you can stuff the blackberries, give them a new look, and put them back in the freezer for later use. Enjoy!

Nutrition:

Carbs: 10 g

Protein: 24 g

Fat: 50 g

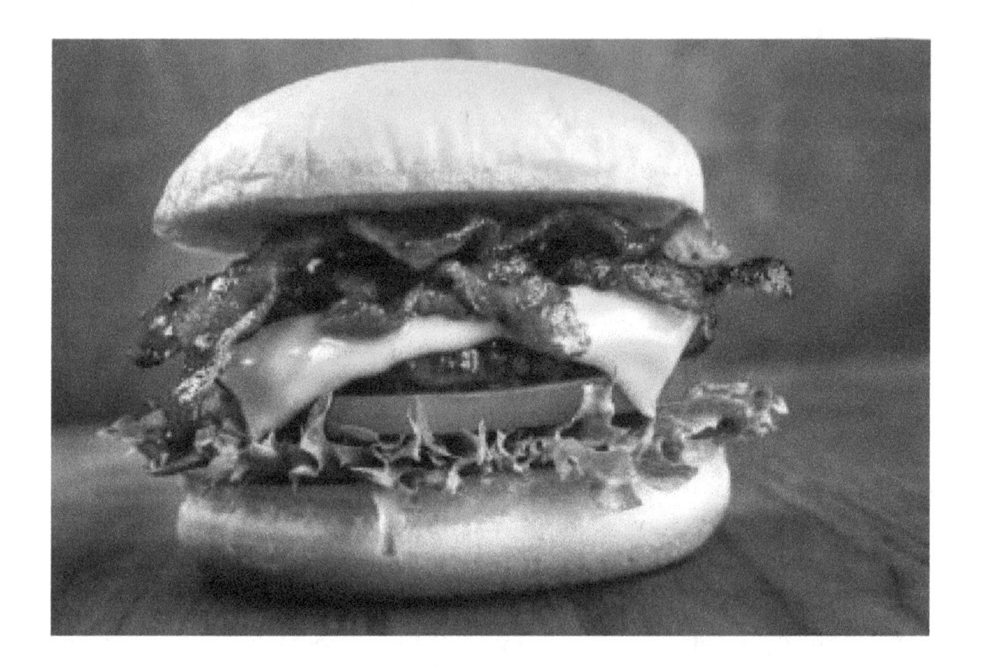

13. Aussie Cheese Fries

Serves: 3

Prep Time: 12-Mins

Cooking Time: 15-Mins

Ingredients:

1-pound frozen chips

6-slices bacon

1½-cups pepper jack cheese

Spicy Ranch Dressing

½-cup Greek yogurt

½-cup sour cream

½-cup buttermilk

2-tablespoons lemon juice

1-teaspoon smoked paprika

1-teaspoon dried dill weed

1-teaspoon dried parsley

1-teaspoon dried thyme

1-teaspoon onion powder

1-teaspoon garlic powder

½-teaspoon dried chives

½-teaspoon cayenne pepper (or more to taste)

½-teaspoon salt

¼-cup mayonnaise

Method:

Prepare the dressing the day before by combining all the ingredients. Place it in a Mason jar in the refrigerator. Preheat the oven and bake the fries according to the directions on the package. Meanwhile, fry the bacon until crispy. Drain it on kitchen paper and chop it finely. When the fries are cooked, sprinkle with cheese and bacon and return them to the oven until the cheese melts. Serve with the spicy ranch dressing. Enjoy!

Nutrition:

Calories: 167.3

Carbs: 27.4 g

Fat: 53.9 g

Protein: 17.2 g

Sodium: 367 mg

14. Panera Cheese And Spinach Egg Soufflé

Serves: 2

Prep Time: 10-Mins

Cooking Time: 5-Mins

Ingredients:

3-ways to start, thawed

3-tablespoons finely chopped

2-teaspoons can be used

1-teaspoon can turn into pepper

5-eggs

2-tablespoons milk

2-possible problems they've had

1/4 cup should be chosen

1/4 cup shredded Monterey Jack cheese

1-tablespoon grated Parmesan cheese

1-8 fold tube Pillsbury Crescent butter flake dough

Cooking spray

1/4 Cup shredded Asiago cheese

1/4 teaspoon of cream puffs

Method:

Preheat the oven to 375 ° F. Combine spinach, artichoke hearts, onion, and purple bell pepper in a small bowl. Add 2 tablespoons of water, cover the bowl with plastic wrap, and put a few containers in the plastic - microwave over high heat for three minutes. Beat four times. Mix in milk, cream, other cheese, Jack cheese, Parmesan, and salt. Indeed, in the story, in the first place, on and in the bubble pepper. Mix the egg aggregate at a high temperature for 30 seconds and then stir it. Do this 4 to 5 more times or until you have a very runny scrambled egg mixture. With this procedure, the eggs are stretched enough so that the dough does not sink into the eggs while also filling. Roll out and rate the new rectangles. Make sure you don't differ the dough from the goal that makes triangles. Instead, compare the work together next to the diagonal perforations so that you have 4-rectangles. Use a few flours on the dough and roll it through the dough with a spinning pin so that each piece of dough comes out well in a six-by-six count. Spray for 4-in-box displays or windows with a specific story. As with any meal with the dough, the dough's same amounts are processed into the same lane. Sprinkle 1-tablespoon of the combination over the entire dish and gently fold the dough over the combination. Beat the remaining egg in a small bowl and brush the beaten egg in each bowl over the dough. Bake for 25 to half an hour or until the dough is brown. Remove from oven and let cool for five minutes, then carefully toss the soufflés from each ramekin and serve hot. Enjoy!

Nutrition:

Carbs: 37 g

Protein: 15 g

Fat: 28 g

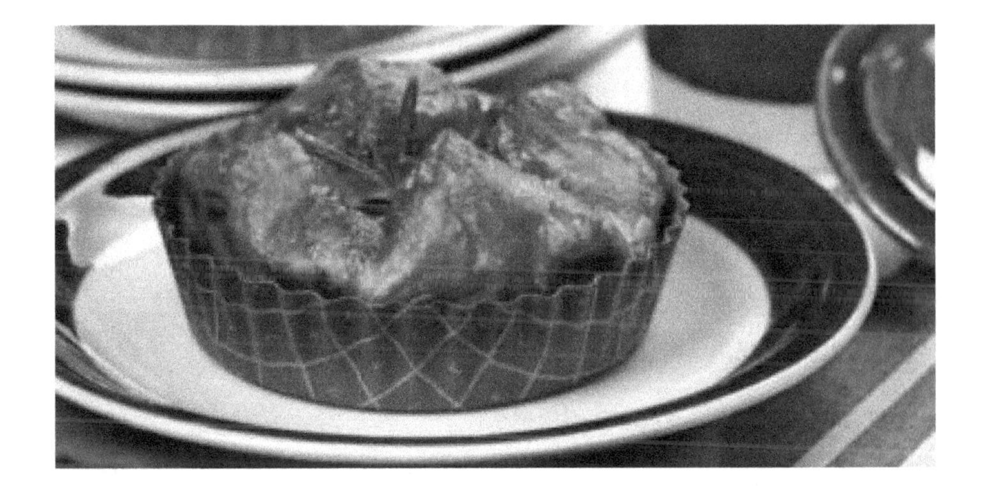

15. Home Baked Potato Soup

Serves: 2

Prep Time: 10-Mins

Cooking Time: 6-Mins

Ingredients:

12 slices of bacon

⅔ cup of margarine

⅔ cup of all-purpose flour

4-large baked potatoes, peeled and cubed

4-green onions, chopped

1-¼ cups of grated Cheddar cheese

1 cup of sour cream

1-teaspoon of salt

1-teaspoon of ground black pepper

7 cups of milk

Method:

Place the bacon in a large, deep skillet. Cook over medium heat until brown. Drain, crumble and set aside. In a stockpot or Dutch oven, soften the margarine over medium heat. Stir the flour until smooth. Fortunately, it starts in no time, which certainly comes to the realization, far away in potatoes and onions. Bring to a boil, stirring frequently. Reduce the heat and within 10 minutes. Mix in cheese, our cream, salt, and pepper. Continue to choose, especially until a decision is made. Enjoy!

Nutrition:

Carbs: 31.4 g

Protein: 8.6 g

16. Cajun Chicken Pasta From Chile

Serves: 4

Prep Time: 13-Mins

Cooking Time: 5-Mins

Ingredients:

2- chicken breasts, boneless and skin

4-teaspoons Cajun seasoning

4-tablespoons of butter or 4-tablespoons of margarine

3 cups of whipped cream

1⁄2 teaspoon of lemon pepper seasoning

1-teaspoon of salt

1-teaspoon of black pepper

8 ounces of penne pasta, cooked and drained

2 Roma tomatoes, diced

1⁄2 cup of Parmesan cheese, shredded fresh, to taste

1⁄4 teaspoon of garlic powder

Method:

Lightly moisten chicken with water. In a large resalable plastic bag, shake the bird and cajun seasoning until the bird is very well covered. In a large frying pan, fry the chicken in 2 tablespoons butter over medium heat, turning over each time. When poultry is halfway through, grab the 2nd skillet, mix heavy cream, 2- tablespoons butter, and the rest of the spices over medium heat, stirring occasionally. When the cream mixture starts to bubble, upload the pasta and turn off the heat. Stir well. When a bird is cooked, place a region on the cutting board and cut it into strips. Spoon pasta and sauce onto large serving dishes (2) and top with the bird, diced tomatoes, and Parmesan cheese. Toss a thick, garlic-like slice of Texas toast on that bad boy. Enjoy!

Nutrition:

Carbs: 26 g

Protein: 28 g

Fat: 17.8 g

17. Mint Chocolate Brownies

Serves: 2

Prep Time: 15-Mins

Cooking Time: 9-Mins

Ingredients:

For the brownie:

180 g dark chocolate

1¼ cup of sugar

100 g unsalted butter

2/3 cup 0000 flour

3-eggs

1-tablespoon of bitter cocoa powder

½ teaspoon of vanilla extract

For the buttercream with mint

100 g unsalted butter

90 g cream cheese

2½ cups of powdered sugar

5-drops of green food coloring

1-pinch of salt

1½ teaspoons of mint extract

½ teaspoon of salt

For cover:

240 g dark chocolate

5-tablespoons of unsalted butter

Method:

Preheat the oven to 180 ° C. Melt the butter and finely chopped dark chocolate in a water bath or microwave, and place aggregate in a large bowl. Add the sugar and mix with a cord beater and add the salt, vanilla extract, sour cocoa powder, and eggs. Finally, add the flour and process with enveloping movements. Thoroughly mix until you get a homogeneous mixture. Pour the brownie instruction onto an 8 "x 11" that was previously protected with molding paper and bake for 25 minutes or until it comes out dry while inserting a toothpick. Let cool on a rack. Put the butter in small cubes in a blender and mix with the cream cheese until you get a creamy result. Add the mint and then the inexperienced edible coloring. Finally, upload the powdered sugar a little at a time. Beat on low speed until a homogeneous aggregate is obtained. Divide the mint buttercream over the bloodless brownie and cover it with paper. Keep in the fridge for 30 minutes. Melt the chocolate and butter in a water bath or the microwave and pour the mint cream on top. Spread with a spatula and put back in the refrigerator for an additional 30 minutes. Enjoy!

18. Rotisserie Chicken

Serves: 5

Prep Time: 12-Mins

Cooking Time: 1-hour

Ingredients:

1⁄4 cup of apple cider vinegar

2-tablespoons of brown sugar

4-fresh cloves of garlic (finely chopped)

1-whole roast chicken

1⁄2 cup of canola oil

Method:

Mix all the elements and pour the poultry into a non-reactive bowl. Let the chook marinate overnight. In the morning, turn the chicken over to marinate the other side. Take the chook out of the refrigerator a few hours later and let it rest for 20 minutes or when it has reached room temperature. I've put this in my view in my idea that it's about half an hour, but you can

do this at 350 for about 45 minutes to an hour or until about a hundred degrees or about a hundred times as many degrees.

Nutrition:

Carbs: 8 g

Protein: 41 g

Fat: 12 g

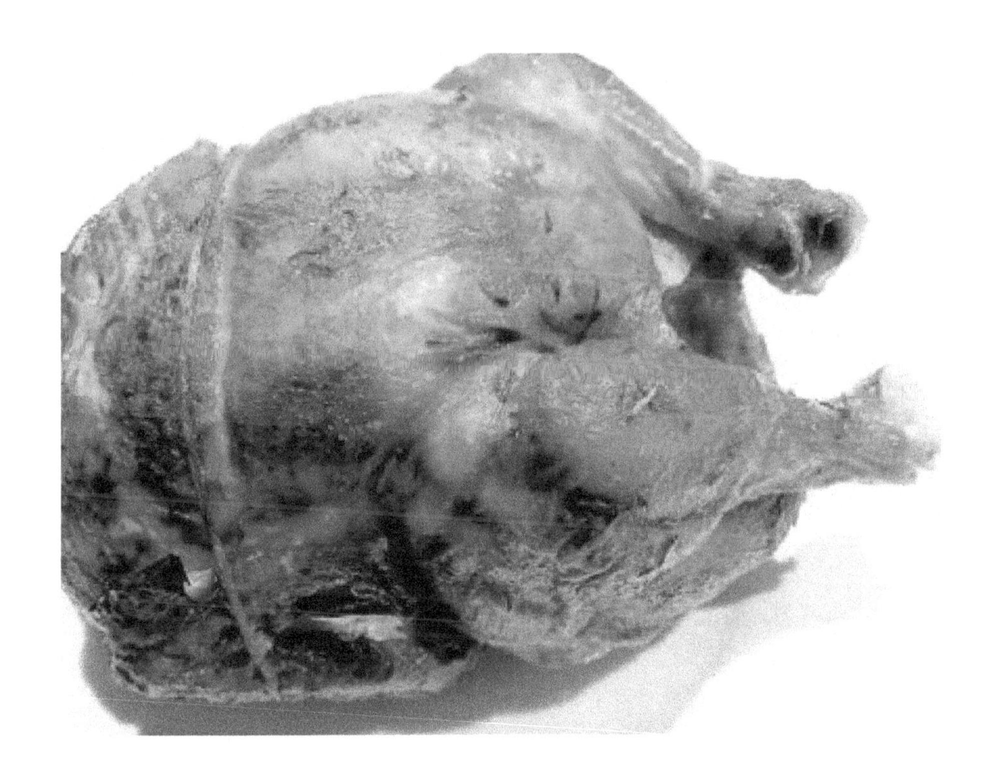

19. Tomatoes Stuffed With Tuna

Serves: 2

Prep Time: 14-Mins

Cooking Time: 15-Mins

Ingredients:

2-cans of water or natural tuna

a large cup of white or brown rice

Mayonnaise c / n

Green olives c / n

Peas or capers c / n

2-carrots

Salt c / n

4-medium tomatoes

Method:

Put a mass of water in a pot and take it to the fireplace. Drain the rice when it boils. Stir with a wooden spoon to keep it from sticking and cook dinner for 20 minutes or until soft. Remove, drain immediately and store in the refrigerator. Cook in a saucepan with water until they soften. Drain and put in a bowl. Add the rice, the two tins of drained tuna, the peas or capers (cooked), and the mayonnaise to taste. Mix everything very well and space to taste. Wash the tomatoes thoroughly and smoke them with a knife and spoon. If you want to use whatever you have chosen for the tomato, cut it into small cubes, mix it with the rice or save it for another recipe. Fill the tomatoes with rice and tuna. Garnish with some mayonnaise in the center and a green olive. Enjoy!

20. Chopped Chicken Salad

Serves: 6

Prep Time: 12-Mins

Cooking Time: 5-Mins

Ingredients:

4-very compact cups of sliced romaine lettuce

2-very small cups of chicory (radicchio) chopped

2-cups of cooked and chopped chicken

8-slices of hard salami OSCAR MAYER Hard salami, chopped

4-ounces (1/2 pc. 8 oz.) Asiago cheese CRACKER BARREL Asiago cheese, chopped

3/4 cup 'on the house' Italian dressing Tuscan style KRAFT Tuscan House

Italian dressing

1 cup ditalini pasta (thimbles), boiled and rinsed

Method:

This salad is simply not satisfying. However, it can also be prepared in advance. Chill up to two hours before serving. Prepare it with robust salami with ground black pepper OSCAR MAYER Cracked Black Pepper Hard Salami. Enjoy!

Nutrition:

Calories: 648

Carbs: 37 g

Protein: 23 g

Fat: 44 g

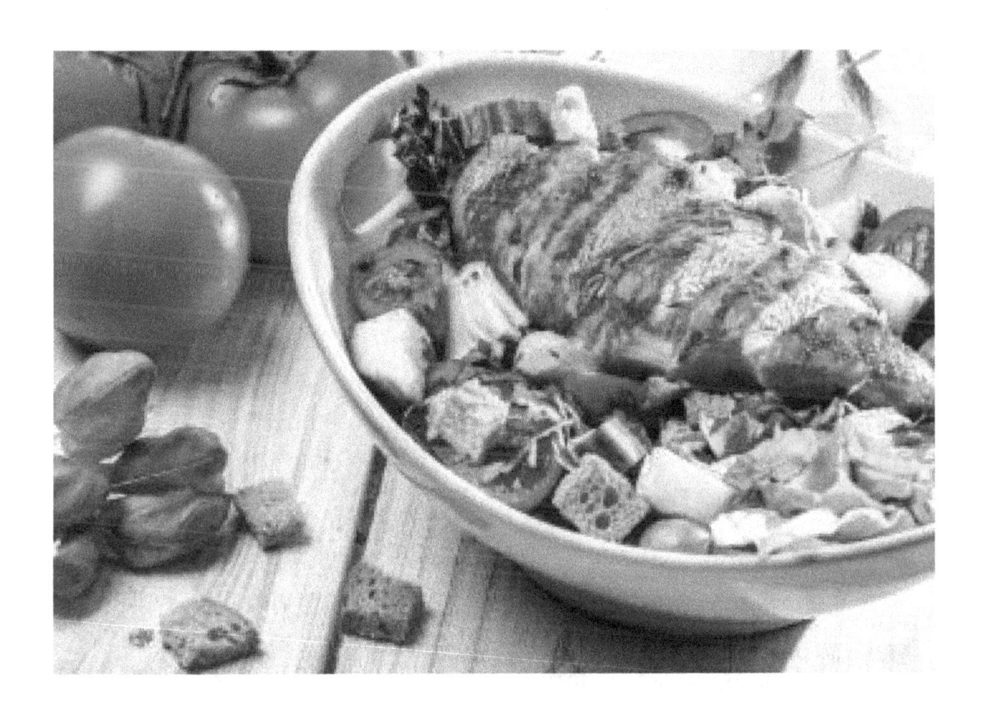

21. Buttermilk Pancakes

Serves: 12-14

Prep Time: 10-Mins

Cooking Time: 4-Mins

Ingredients:

2 cups of non-sifted flour

2-teaspoons of baking powder

1-teaspoon of salt

3-tablespoons of sugar

2-⅓ cups of low-fat buttermilk

Butter for cooking

2-eggs

Method:

Preheat a baking sheet or large skillet to 350 ° F. Place a buttered piece close to the pan; you can make it butter before preparing any pancake. Beat the eggs and buttermilk in a medium bowl until well blended. Beat in the flour, baking soda, sugar, and salt. Beat thoroughly until well blended. Prepare the skillet by rubbing the butter in a circle in the center, then adding about ½ cup of batter. Divide the batter until it forms an even circle. When the pancake surface becomes fizzy, turn over and cook on the other side until you can't see any wet spots on the edges. Repeat with the remaining batter, making sure to sprinkle the skillet before starting each pancake. Serve with your favorite syrup or fruit. Enjoy!

Nutrition:

Calories: 110

Carbs: 34 g

Total fat: 6 g

Protein: 6 g

22. Cheese Broccoli

Serves: 4

Prep Time: 5-Mins

Cooking Time: 15-Mins

Ingredients:

2-tablespoons butter

2-tablespoons flour

1-cup whipped cream

½-cup milk

¼-teaspoon salt

¼-teaspoon black pepper

½-teaspoon paprika powder

½-teaspoon garlic powder

½-teaspoon ground mustard

8-ounces crisp cheddar cheese, shredded (plus more for topping)

6–8 cups fresh broccoli florets, rinsed

¼-teaspoon cayenne powder

Method:

Preheat the oven to 375 ° F and coat 6 (10-ounces or so) casseroles with cooking spray. Melt the butter in a large, heavy-bottomed pan or a Dutch oven. Beat in the flour. Cook and stir until the roux turns a light golden color. Gradually beat in the cream and milk until smooth. Add the spices. Cook over medium heat until the sauce thickens. Stir in cheese until melted. Meanwhile, steam the broccoli in a separate pan until bright green but still crispy. Add the broccoli to the white sauce and stir to coat. Spoon the broccoli and white sauce into the prepared dishes. Top with more cheese. Bake for 3-5 minutes, until the cheese melts on top and the edges are hot and bubbly. Enjoy!

Nutrition:

Calories: 767.3

Fat: 52.9 g

Carbs: 57.4 g

Protein: 17.2 g

Sodium: 367 mg

23. Apple Bee Lean Quesadilla

Serves: 2

Prep Time: 16-Mins

Cooking Time: 5-Mins

Ingredients:

1⁄2 ounce shortening

2 (12 inches) flour tortillas

2-tablespoons of hot chipotle sauce

4-ounces grilled chicken (seasoning optional)

4-ounces of sour cream

2-ounces of green onions

4-ounces of salsa

1-cup of lettuce, shredded

Method:

Brush one facet of each tortilla with a cut. Place a tortilla on the work floor with the short side down. Divide the chipotle sauce evenly on a tortilla. If the chicken was no longer freshly grilled, then microwave the chicken for about 45 seconds, then gently spread over the sauce's top on the tortilla. Divide Quesa Filling evenly over the poultry. Then cover with the other tortilla and shorten the facet. Bake on the baking sheet or in any pan frivolously on each side until the inner filling is thoroughly heated. Use grated lettuce, sour cream, inexperienced onion, and salsa as side dishes. I like to put crumbled bacon on top. Enjoy!

Nutrition:

Carbs: 84 g

Protein: 48 g

Fat: 30 g

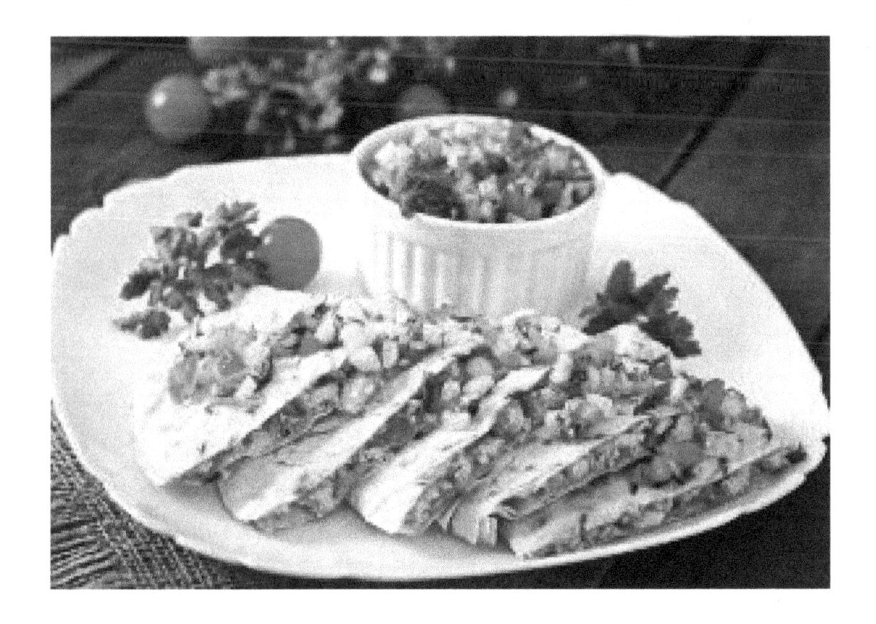

24. Sonic's Supersonic Burrito

Serves: 2

Prep Time: 10-Mins

Cooking Time: 5-Mins

Ingredients:

1 1/2 cups Tater Tots

1-pound ground says

1/2 pound bacon

6-months ago

4-different types of milk, depending on the use

10-eggs

and pepper

1-jalapeno pepper disappears

6-flour tartllas

1/2 cup made a different choice

Method:

Preheat the oven to 350 degrees. Spray a baking sheet with non-stick cooking spray and place the Tater Tots on the baking sheet. Bake for about 22 to 25 minutes. While the little tots are in the oven, cook the sausage in a skillet over medium heat until it is nicely browned. Drink says about towels and chooses by all other means to help keep the

heat in as you can still choose the shortest. You can cook the bacon in the pan in which you chose the food. Cook the bacon until good. Absorb from the pan and enjoy the best towels. Sonic serves their burrito with a cheese dish. Cubic the 6 oz of American cheese
and place in a small pot over low heat and upload 2 tablespoons from milk. Melt them, stirring freely. The mixture and the flavor will form a cheese sauce. Once your chosen sauce has been chosen, turning off the burner and leaving the tray on the plate, the remaining heat will keep the sauce runny even as you prepare the eggs. In a medium bowl, place the eggs with the last 2-tablespoons of milk. Spray a non-stick skillet with non-stick cooking spray. Upload the egg and milk combination over medium heat - a few times with a small amount and a blank paper pinch. Gently stir ste ste as they pepare iner. Only they can be put off by the heat. Expect to make and make up for them about 60 times. Assemble these by dividing the eggs, sausage, potato cakes, bacon, and cheese sauce over the tortillas. If you want to upload some jalapeno slices to the burritos, do so; if you want to, upload a little cheddar cheese before stuffing the blackberries. If you can, fill up the blackberries, and pack them up in one sitting and use the freezer so you can use them again later. Enjoy!

Nutrition:

Carbs: 10 g

Protein: 24 g

25. Chicken Tortilla Soup

Serves: 2

Prep Time: 10-Mins

Cooking Time: 5-Mins

Ingredients:

1-chicken fillet; chopped into small pieces

½ cup sweet corn

1 cup onion, chopped

3-tablespoons fresh cilantro, chopped

1 cup chicken stock

1-can diced peppers and tomatoes (8 grams)

Colby jack cheese to taste

1-splash of lime juice in an individual bowl

Tortilla chips to taste

1 cup of water

Avocado to taste

Method:

In a large, deep saucepan over medium heat, combine the chicken stock with water, onion, chili, and tomatoes, corn and cilantro; bring the mixture to a boil, stirring occasionally. Add the chicken pieces; stir well, and reduce heat to low. Cook for a few minutes until the chicken is cooked. Add tortilla chips, followed by avocado and cheese to taste in serving dishes. Add soup and a squeeze of lime to the bowls. Serve hot. Enjoy!

Nutrition:

Calories: 305

Total fat: 5 g

Carbs: 27 g

Protein: 34 g

Sodium: 1024 mg

26. Three Applebee Cheese Chicken Penne

Serves: 2

Prep Time: 10-Mins

Cooking Time: 5-Mins

Ingredients:

1-teaspoon of fresh basil leaf; thin sliced

2-small Roma tomatoes; cut into pieces

1-clove of garlic; pressed

1/4 teaspoon of salt

1/2 teaspoon of olive oil

1 pound chicken breast

2-tablespoons of lemon juice

1/2 teaspoon of Italian seasoning

5-buttons mushroms; Loss

1-tablespon purple onion; a lot less (optional)

1-jar of garlic alfredo sauce

2-ounces provolone cheese; shredded or chopped small

2-ounces grated parmesan cheese

2-ounces mozzarella cheese; choppped small or shredded

2-teaspoons of olive oil

1/2 pound of pasta; according to the directions below

1-tablespoon of olive oil

Method:

2T just once, 1 T of olive oil and an Italian view, take another chicken and place in a plastic container or Marinator. (instead of an amount sealed within hours) marinate for 30 minutes to several hours. Also, start bruschetta aggregate. Simply mix everything and cover it in the refrigerator until dinner is ready to serve. Meanwhile, heat 2-teaspoons of olive oil over medium heat in a heavy skillet and cook the mushrooms and onions until tender. Add the empty jar of Alfredo sauce to the pan and add the drained cooked pasta. Chook is ready. Cut thick or thin and upload to the skillet. Heat the skillet contents until they are quite bubbly, then upload the cheeses and mix properly until blended and blended. Serve pasta dishes and top with bruschetta mix and some garlic bread or sticks, making a great meal! Enjoy!

Nutrition:

Carbs: 91 g

Protein: 57 g

Fat: 46 g

27. Chili's Melted Lava Cake

Serves: 2

Prep Time: 10-Mins

Cooking Time: 5-Mins

Ingredients:

1-14-ounce can have sweetened condensed milk

1-bag of 12 ounces plus

1-cup semi-sweet chocolate chips, divided

4-tablespoons unsalted butter

1-teaspoon pure vanilla extract

1-pinch salt

1-packet fudge cake mix

3-large eggs

½-cup sour cream

½-cup canola oil

Cooking spray with non-stick coating

1-cup milk chocolate chips

¼-cup coconut oil

Vanilla ice cream

Caramel syrup

1-cup milk

Method:

Make hot fudge by adding condensed milk, one bag of chocolate chips, butter, vanilla, and salt to a saucepan over medium heat, stirring frequently. After cooking, it continues for about 2 minutes. Turn off the heat, but keep stirring the mixture for 1 minute more. Set aside to cool. Combine cake mix, eggs, sour cream, milk, and oil in a bowl. Put aside. Coat a melted cake tin or cupcake tin with non-stick cooking spray and pour the batter into each mold. Leave about ¼ mold without batter. Bake according to the packaging. Then invert cakes to form a volcano shape and let them cool. Carefully cut some cake from the center of each into a cone, but not all the

way through. Pour cooled hot fudge into the hole. Take the cut cake pan, cut a thin slice on the main part, and place it like a cap over the hot fudge. While the cake is cooling, prepare magic shells by microwaving a bowl of coconut oil and the remaining chocolate chips in 30-second intervals, stirring after each interval until melted. Wait to cool down. Serve cakes on a plate and top with frozen dessert, followed by caramel, then magic bowl. Enjoy!

Nutrition:

Calories: 350

Carbs: 28 g

Total fat: 26 g

Saturated fat: 5 g

Fiber: 2 g,

Protein: 6 g

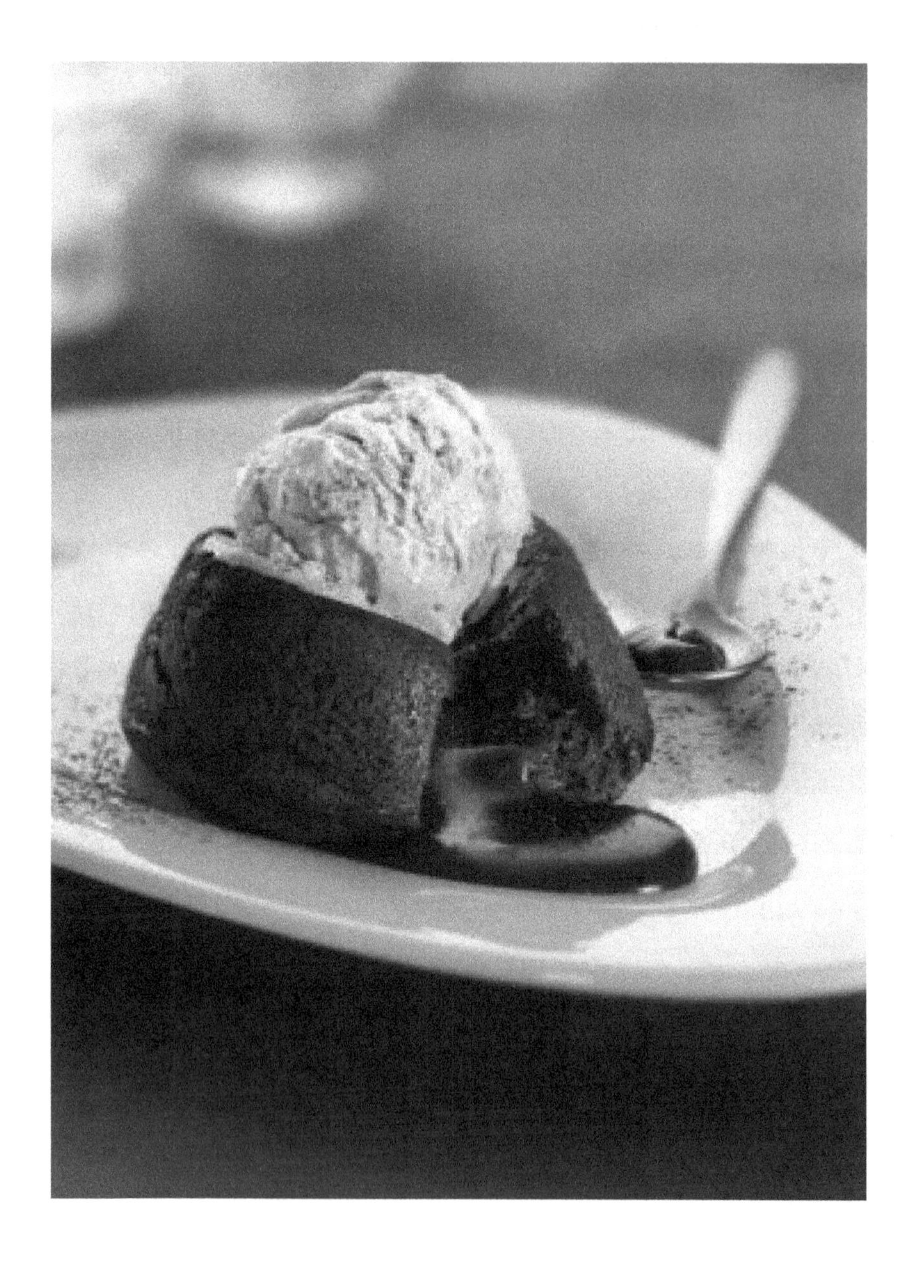

28. Cracker Barrel Chicken And Dumplings

Serves: 4

Prep Time: 20-Mins

Cooking Time: 45-Mins

Ingredients:

2-cups of flour

1/2 teaspoon of baking powder

2-tablespoons of butter

1 cup of milk

2 liters of chicken stock

3 cups of cooked chicken

1-pinch of salt

Method:

Place the flour, baking powder, and salt in a bowl. Cut the butter into the dry substances with a fork or pastry knife. Stay in the milk, mix with a bottle to the end of a ball. Sprinkle a piece of the surface with flour. You will need a rolling pin and something to cut the dumplings with. I would like to request a pizza cutter. I also like to use a small spatula to lift the dumplings off the cutting surface. Roll out the dough thinly with a heavily floured rolling pin. Dip your cutter in flour and cut the dumplings into squares about 2x2 inches each. It's okay for them now, not to be exact. Just look at it. Some can be bigger, some smaller, and some can be funny shaped. Cook them for about 15 to 20 minutes or until they don't taste doughy. Add the cooked chicken to the pan and serve. Enjoy!

Nutrition:

Carbs: 55 g

Protein: 37 g

Fat: 9 g

29. California Pizza

Serves: 6

Prep Time: 20-Mins

Cooking Time: 10-Mins

Ingredients:

1-tablespoon of cornmeal

1-piece (1 pound) frozen pizza dough, thawed

1 cup of grated mozzarella cheese

1 cup ready-to-eat grilled chicken fillet strips

4-bacon strips, cooked and crumbled

2 cups of grated romaine

1 cup of fresh arugula

1-tablespoon of lemon juice

1-teaspoon of lemon zest

1/2 teaspoon of pepper

1-medium tomato, thinly sliced

1-medium ripe avocado, peeled and sliced

1/4 cup loosely packed basil leaves, chopped

1/4 cup of mayonnaise

Method:

Preheat the oven to 450 °. Grease a 14-in. Pizza; sprinkle with cornmeal. On a smooth surface, do a 13-in. Sure. Transfer to organized pan; slightly raise the edges. Sprinkle with cheese, poultry, and bacon. Bake until crust is gently browned for 10-12 minutes. Meanwhile, place the romaine and arugula in a large bowl. In a small bowl, add mayonnaise, lemon juice, lemon zest, and pepper. Pour over the lettuce; toss to coat. Arrange overheated pizza. Top with tomato, avocado, and basil. Serve immediately. Enjoy!

Nutrition:

Carbs: 59 g

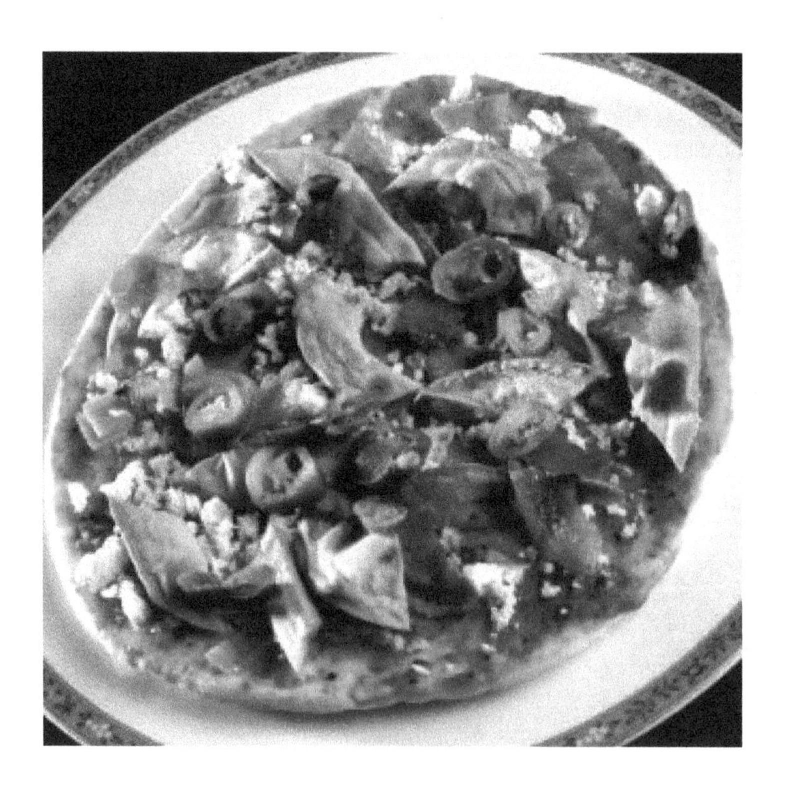

30. Shrimp Tempura

Serves: 2

Prep Time: 20-Mins

Cooking Time: 10-Mins

Ingredients:

1/2 kg of clean shrimps

Garlic and salt for flavoring shrimp

5-tablespoons of flour

1-red seasonal envelope or seasonal for fish oil for frying

4-whole eggs

Method:

Season the smooth shrimp with garlic and salt and set aside. Beat whole eggs until soft, add a pinch of salt, the spices, and the flour, and beat with a fork until smooth. Gradually dip the shrimp in this batter and fry them in warm oil. When browning the dough with a slotted spoon and drain on absorbent kitchen paper. Serve warm as it tastes, or perhaps with white rice and shrimp sauce. Enjoy!

31. Sonic's Supersonic Burrito

Serves: 2

Prep Time: 10-Mins

Cooking Time: 5-Mins

Ingredients:

50-potato cakes, frozen

1 pound of breakfast sausage patties

8-large eggs, beaten

2-tablespoons half and half

Salt and pepper to taste

8-flour tortillas of 15 cm

1½ cups of cheddar cheese, grated

1-medium onion, diced

½ cup pickled jalapeño peppers, sliced

3-Roma tomatoes, sliced

Salsa

1-tablespoon of butter

Method:

Cook potato cakes according to package directions, but cook them so they are slightly crispy. Put aside. Cook sausage patties in a pan. Divide into large clumps until brown. Add eggs, half and half, salt, and pepper in a bowl. Beat until well blended. Heat butter in a pan over medium heat. Pour the egg mixture and occasionally stir into scrambled eggs. Remove from heat. Microwave tortillas until warm but still soft. Then, in a vertical line down the center, add cheddar cheese, eggs, cooked sausage, potato cakes, onions, jalapeños, and tomato. Fold the ingredients using the outer flaps of the tortilla. Repeat with the remaining ingredients and tortillas. Serve hot with salsa. Enjoy!

Nutrition:

Calories: 636

Carbs: 39 g

Total fat: 40 g

Saturated fat: 16 g

Sugar: 4 g

Fiber: 3 g

Protein: 28 g

Sodium: 1381 mg

32. Burger & Sandwich

Serves: 1

Prep Time: 15-Mins

Cooking Time: 10-Mins

Ingredients:

Another oil cooking spray

1-pound lean or ery lean ground beef

1-new text

1/4 cup onion inced

3-differences from the Cheddar choice

6-small sandwiches

1.5 Tablespoons ketchup

1-Tablespoon weweet relish

1-tablespoon of pickle juice

1-tablespoon of finely chopped onion

1/8 teaspoon of garlic powder

1/8 teaspoon of paprika

1/8 teaspoon of onion powder

1/8 teaspoon of mustard powder

1/2 cup light mayo

Method:

Preheat the oven to 350 levels F. Provide the bottom of a 13x9 inch baking pan with even more oil spray. Save the soil and fly directly to the bottom of the previous baking sheet. Bake ground pork in the oven for 20 minutes or until the temperature is 160 levels F. While the beef is cooking, prepare the sauce: put all components in a small bowl and mix until combined. When beef is cooked, remove it from the pan and cut it into 12 of the same squares. Place the lettuce on the bottom of a sliding roll. Top with a beef patty. Then add cheese (half of a slice is good). Top cheese with any other Patty and then pickles. Divide the sauce over the top of the sliding bun and add a pinch of onion. Enjoy!

Nutrition:

Carbs: 14.4 g

Protein: 19.9 g

Fat: 8 g

33. Olive Garden Salad And Creamy Dressing

Serves: 4

Prep Time: 15-Mins

Cooking Time: 25-Mins

Ingredients:

1-pack of Good Seasonings Italian Dressing

ingredients needed to make dressing; oil, water, and vinegar

½ teaspoon of dried Italian herbs

½ teaspoon of table salt

½ tsp sugar

¼ tsp garlic powder

½ tbsp mayonnaise

¼ cup of olive oil

2-tbsp white vinegar

1 ½ tbsp water

¼ tsp black pepper

Method:

Prepare Good Seasonings Italian Seasonings Dressing as it says on the back of the package (mix with oil, water, and vinegar in the dimensions on the package). Once prepared to pour into a medium bowl, add any additional substances indexed above (starting with dried Italian herbs). Mix all the elements with a whisk until well blended. Serve with your favorite salads. Enjoy!

Nutrition:

Carbs: 8.9 g

Protein: 1.1 g

Fat: 10.2 g

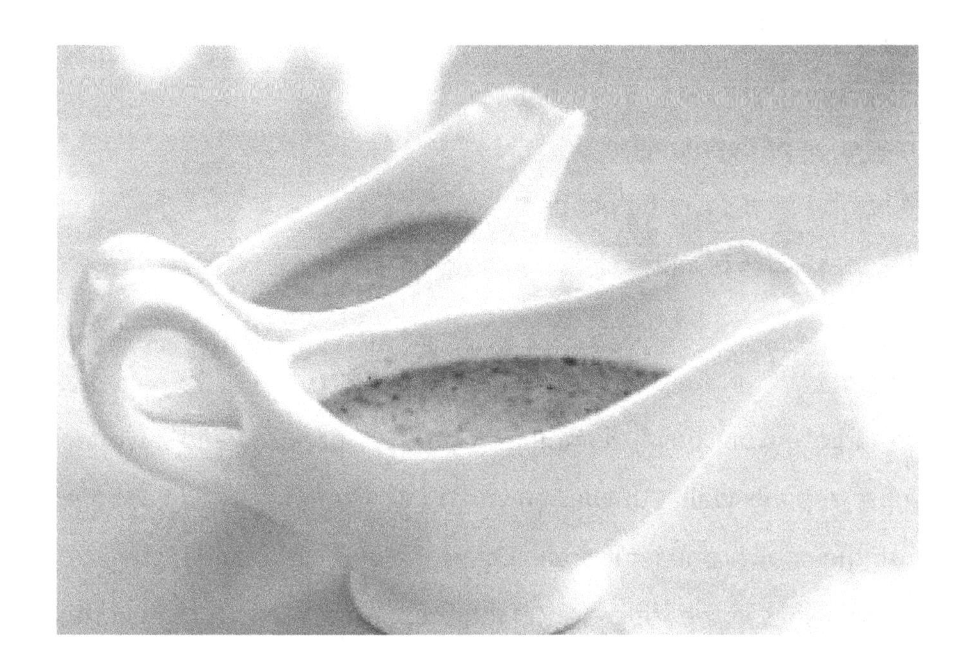

34. Hot N 'Spicy Buffalo Wings

Serves: 2

Prep Time: 10-Mins

Cooking Time: 5-Mins

Ingredients:

Cut 5 pounds of chicken wings into half

2 cups of whole wheat flour

1 cup all-purpose flour

1-teaspoon of paprika

1/4 teaspoon of cayenne pepper

2 1/2 teaspoons of salt

Method:

In a large mixing bowl, combine flour, salt, paprika, and cayenne pepper and mix well. Cut chicken wings into drumettes and flappers. Wash the poultry and let it drain. Cover the bird with flour aggregate; put bird wings in the fridge for 90 minutes. Spread the chicken in the flour mixture; Put chicken wings in the refrigerator for 90 minutes. If equipped to fry chicken wings, heat the oil to reach 375. Place the poultry pieces in heated oil, but do not compress them. Fry the chicken wings until golden brown. Remove from oil and drain. When all the wings are cooked, place them in a huge bowl. Add Hot Sauce aggregate and mix well. Use a fork or tongs to place chicken pieces on a serving platter. Serve now and with plenty of kitchen paper. Enjoy!

Nutrition:

Carbs: 44 g

Protein: 44 g

Fat: 33 g

35. Chili's Chili

Serves: 2

Prep Time: 10-Mins

Cooking Time: 6-Mins

Ingredients:

For Chile:

4-pounds ground chuck - ground for chili

1½ cups yellow onions, chopped

1-tablespoon cooking oil

3¼ plus 1 cup of water

1-tablespoon Masa Harina

16 ounces tomato sauce

For Chili Spice Blend:

1-tablespoon paprika

½ cup of chili powder

1-teaspoon ground black pepper

1-teaspoon cayenne pepper or to taste

1/8 cup salt

1-teaspoon garlic powder

1/8 cup of ground cumin

Method:

Mix the whole chili seasoning ingredients in a small bowl; still, mix until thoroughly mixed. Now, in a 6-quart stockpot over medium heat; place and cook the meat until brown; drain. In the meantime, combine the chili spice mix in addition to the spaghetti sauce and 3¼ cups of water in the bowl; stir the ingredients well until well blended. Add the chili spice liquid to the browned meat; stir well, and bring the mixture to a boil over medium heat. In a large frying pan over medium heat; Heat 1 tablespoon of the vegetable oil and fry the onions for a few minutes until translucent. Add the fried onions to the chili. Reduce heat and simmer for an hour, stirring after every 10 to 15 minutes. Combine the masa Harina with the remaining water in a separate bowl; mix well. Add the chili stockpot and cook for another 10 minutes. Enjoy!

Nutrition:

Calories: 205

Carbs: 27 g

Total fat: 5 g

Protein: 34 g

Sodium: 1024 mg

36. Kung Pao Spaghetti California Pizza Chicken

Serves: 4

Prep Time: 13-Mins

Cooking Time: 5-Mins

Ingredients:

1⁄2 cups of chicken stock

2-tablespoons of cornstarch

3⁄4 cup of soy sauce

1⁄2 cup of dry sherry

3-tablespoons of red chili paste with garlic

1⁄4 cup of sugar

2-tablespoons of red wine vinegar

2-tablespoons of toasted sesame oil

2-proteins

2-tablespoons of cornstarch

1⁄2 teaspoon of salt

1 lb spaghetti

1⁄2-part olive oil, plus

1-pound skinless note, cut into 3/4-inch cubes

10-15, while the choices you make can find certain parts

1 cup to date dry peanuts

1⁄4 cup can reduce

3-choices for certain

things, greetings, and whites

2-tablespoons olives oil

Method:

In a medium saucepan, beat the poultry inventory and cornstarch together until the cornstarch is completely dissolved. Stir in all ingredients for the closing sauce and bring to a boil over medium heat. Repair the heat, and simmer is thick enough to dial it again from a break, 15 to twenty minutes. Set. In a mixing bowl, use a whisk to stir the egg whites, cornflour, and salt together well; be careful not to beat them to foam any longer. Put aside. Bring a huge pot of salted water to a boil. Add the pasta and make dinner al dente, eight to ten minutes. Meanwhile, in a large non-stick frying pan over high heat, heat the olive oil for about 1 minute. Add the chicken pieces to the protein cornstarch mixture to select them. Take time to start, add the chosen bird to the pan and cook the dinner like a stable pancake until the egg aggregate solidifies; Then, using a large spatula, carefully turn the poultry pieces together and observe the characteristics with a wood carving. Gently stir the Chinese peppers and roasted peanuts into the pan. As soon as they turn dark in color, after no more than 1 minute, stir in the garlic and spring onions. Once the garlic starts to brown, after no more than 30 seconds, upload the Kung Pao sauce and stir to find the ingredients. When the pasta is ready, drain it nicely and mix well with the sauce in a large mixing or serving bowl. Serve family fashion or transfer to individual serving dishes, arranging the chicken, vegetables, and peppers. Enjoy!

Nutrition:

Carbs: 129 g

Protein: 57 g

Fat: 44 g

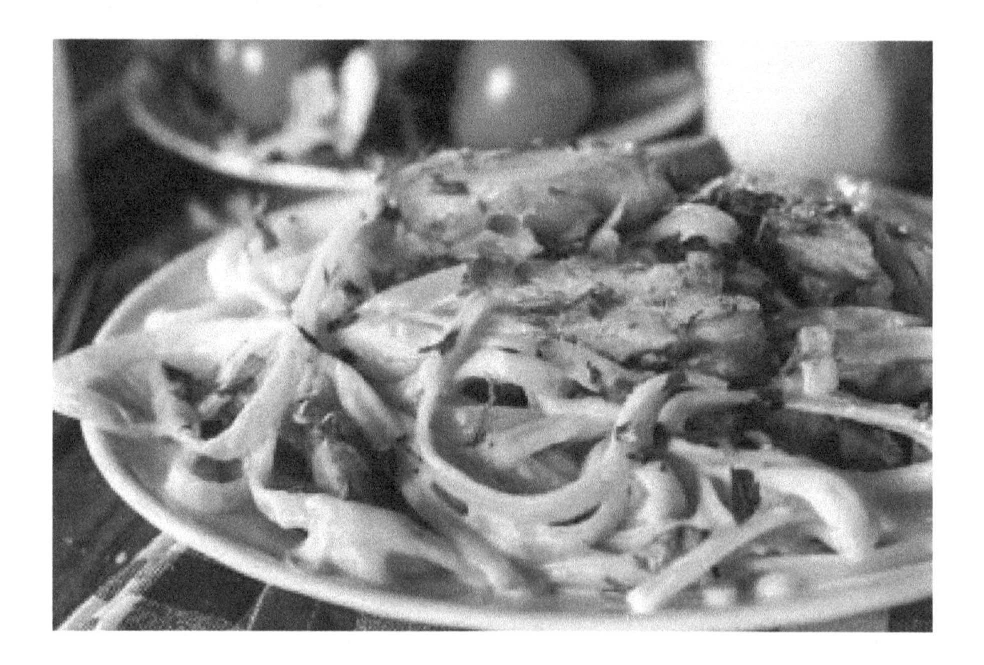

37. Blueberry Cheesecake

Serves: 3

Prep Time: 10-Mins

Cooking Time: 6-Mins

Ingredients:

For the basics:

240 g crunchy sweet biscuits

120 g butter

For the cheesecake

3/4 of Philadelphia cream cheese

180 ml cream or milk cream

150 g of sugar

100 g fresh blueberries

20 g cornstarch

1-egg yolk

1-tablespoon of vanilla extract

2-eggs

For cover:

150 g white chocolate

80 ml cream or milk cream

Method:

Process the cookies and mix them with the melted butter until you get a paste. Place at the lowest point of a removable mold with a diameter of 20 cm and a height of 5 to 7 cm. Spread over the bottom, flatten with the back of a spoon or the palm of your hand, and reserve. Mix the liquid with the filter until there are no more lumps. Add the yolk and eggs. Mix the cornstarch with the cream or milk cream, blueberries, and vanilla extract. Turn the instruction over the dough. Bake for 45-50 minutes at 170 ° C. Leave to cool in the oven. Chop the white chocolate and set it aside. Heat the cream or milk cream in a pan and add the cream to the chopped white chocolate. Mix and, while melted, unfold at the blueberry cheesecake once cold. Enjoy!

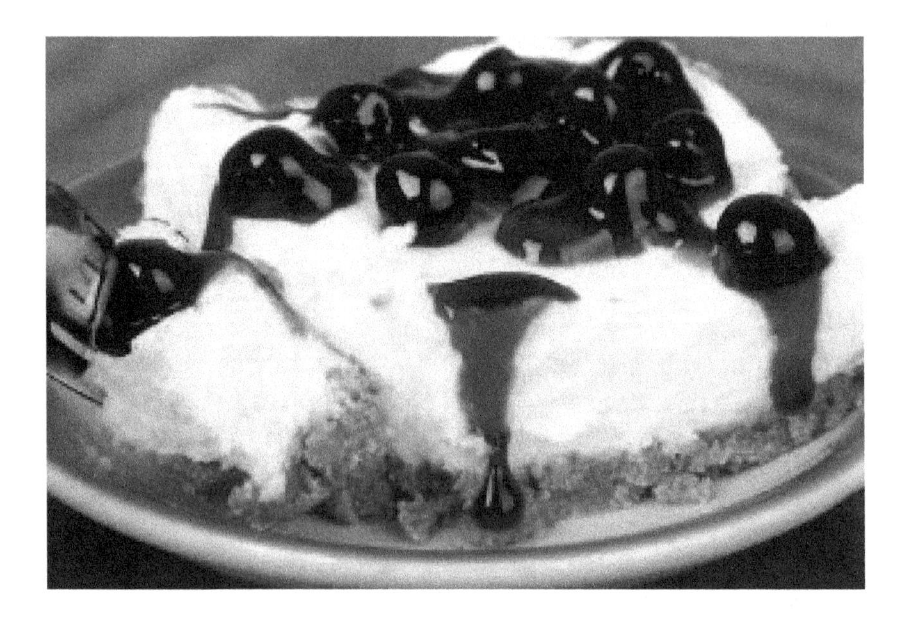

38. Salmon Gravlax

Serves: 6

Prep Time: 16-Mins

Cooking Time: 25-Mins

Ingredients:

2-salmon fillets of 1 kilo each, without skin

¼ cup of vodka

1/3 cup of sugar

1-tablespoon of ground black pepper

¼ cup of chopped dill

1/3 cup of fine sea salt

Method:

Collect the salmon gravlax components. Rinse and dry the salmon fillets well. Use pliers or pliers to remove the spines if necessary. Sprinkle the salmon lightly with the vodka. In a small bowl, mix sugar, pleasant sea salt, and black pepper on the floor. Divide the aggregate into three identical parts in the bowl. Place half the 0.33 of the curing aggregate on a rimmed baking tray. Add a skinless salmon fillet to the mixture and divide one-third over the aggregate at the fillet. Divide the opposite 1/2 of the third over the second steak and sprinkle with chopped dill. Place the second fillet on top of the first and sprinkle the sealing aggregate over the top salmon's skin. Cover the tray with foil and place a wooden plate on top of the covered fish. Cover with a heavy pot and refrigerate for at least 12 hours. Remove from the refrigerator and dispose of the collected liquid in the container. Return the salmon to the refrigerator for 12 hours. The fish is already healed, and you could serve it. However, it continues to benefit from every other 12 to 24 hours of cooling. Enjoy!

Nutrition:

Calories: 238

Fats: 12 g

Carbs: 3 g

Protein: 27 g

39. Pizza Hut Cavatina

Serves: 2

Prep Time: 14-Mins

Cooking Time: 15-Mins

Ingredients:

Thinly slice 1/2 pound of peppers

1/4 pound of spiral pasta

1-green pepper chopped

1/4-pound Shell noodles

Cut 1-onion into thin slices

8-ounces of grated mozzarella

1/2-pound hamburger brown

8 grams of grated Parmesan cheese

1/2-pound Italian sausage brown

32 grams of spaghetti sauce

1/4 pound of pasta

Method:

Cook noodles in the course of the package. Heat the sauce and mix it with the hamburger and the fried sausage. Sprinkled with Pam cooking spray, noodles, and sauce layers in 11 X 13 pan. Layer pepperoni, green peppers, and onions, mushrooms, and cheese.

Make about 3-layers of cheese and cover with it. Baking for about forty-five minutes in 350 states or until the cheese is melted. Enjoy!

Nutrition:

Calories: 467

Carbs: 36 g

Protein: 24 g

Fat: 24 g

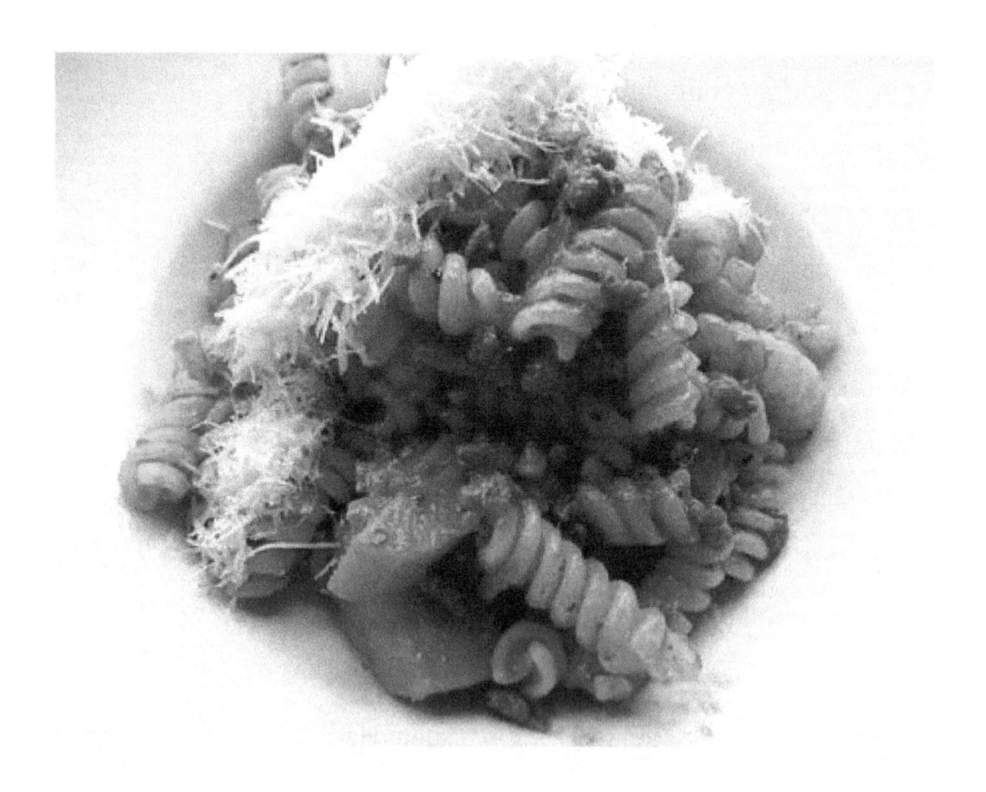

40. Chilis Southwest Egg Rolls

Prep Time: 15-Mins

Cooking Time: 25-Mins

Serves: 4

Ingredients:

8-oz chicken breast

1-teaspoon of vegetable olive oil is fine

1-tablespoon of vegetable olive oil is fine

1/4 cup chopped red bell pepper

1/4 cup chopped scallions

1/2 cup of frozen corn

1/2 cup canned black beans, ready and drained

1/4 cup frozen spinach, thawed and drunk

2-examples of pickled jalapeno pepper, prepared

3/4 cup grated Monterey Jack cheese

8/7 inch flour tortillas

1/4 cup pureed fresh avocados (about half an avocado)

1-pack of Ranch Dressing Mix

1/2 cup of milk

1/2 cup of mayonnaise

2-tablespoons of chopped tomatoes

1-tablespoon of chopped onions

1-teaspoon of taco seasoning

Method:

Season with salt and black pepper to the poultry. Brush the chicken breast with olive oil. Grill on a grill over medium heat. Cook on each side for five to seven minutes. Cut the chicken into small pieces. Set the poultry aside. Fry until tender red pepper. Refer to the total of the green onion, rice, black beans, spinach, and pickled jalapenos. Attach the seasoning for the taco through the sun. Place the tortillas in the same amounts of filings, identical amounts of chicken, and drizzle with cheese. Fold and roll up the ends of the tortilla. Make sure the tortillas are very tight to roll. Now defend the pin with toothpicks. We grow enough vegetable oil in a large pot to cover the back of the pan 10 cm. Heat to 350 ° C. Deep fries the egg rolls until golden brown. It should take seven to eight minutes. When extracting gold from oil, grow it on a wire rack. Prepare a mayonnaise container, half cup of ranch dressing mix, and a half cup of buttermilk. Remove the total of 1/4 cup of mashed avocado. Pump the combination into a blender until the sauce is blended. Enjoy!

Nutrition:

Calories: 502

Carbs: 42g

Protein: 19g

Conclusion

And here we come to the end. Thanks to this cookbook you are now aware of all the ingredients that go into each recipe, but you will also save money!

We all love to eat out; whether it's with a friend or another, there's something enjoyable and exciting about it.

However, you'll agree with me that even though we want to eat out all the time, preparing homemade meals is always the best option, not only because you know the ingredients of the food, but because you save money.

Thanks to this cookbook you can replicate the most famous and tasty dishes from restaurants, even if you are not a professional cook.

Not to mention the hassle of driving, standing in line, and paying way more than the actual cost is more than enough reason to try making your favorites at home.

I imagine you were surprised at how easy some of them are to prepare. Save your time, energy, and expense out of going to a restaurant with these amazing copycat recipes!

You're craving your favorite restaurant meal, but not the drive, the wait, or the bill. Now you can make it yourself! Home cooks are serving up their best copycat recipes, right here.

Save some money by not having to hire a babysitter, and stay in comfy clothes at home!

Enjoy and have fun!

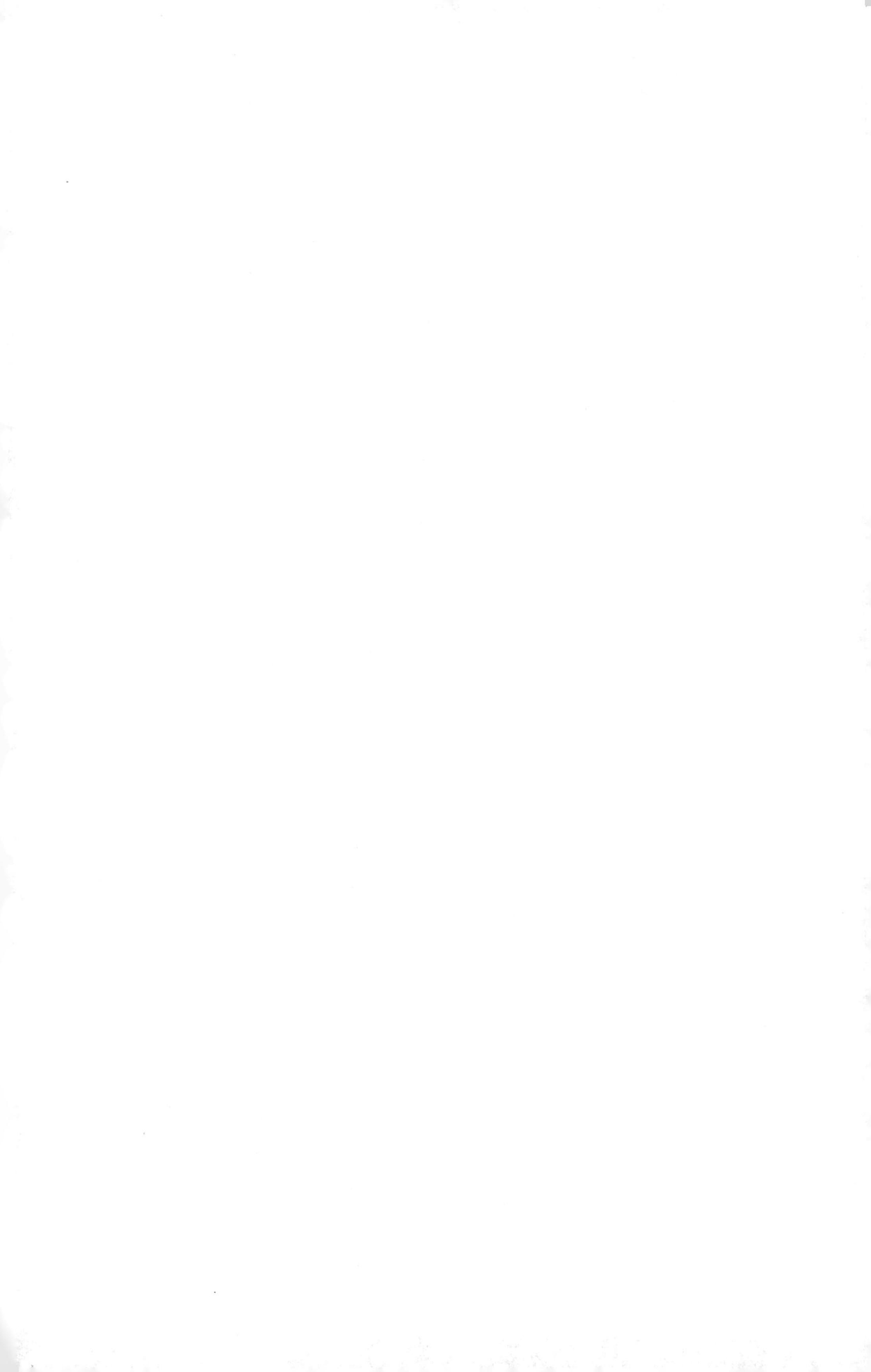

CPSIA information can be obtained
at www.ICGtesting.com
Printed in the USA
BVHW061120200421
605389BV00003B/494

9 781801 827775